YOUR KNOWLEDGE HAS VALUE

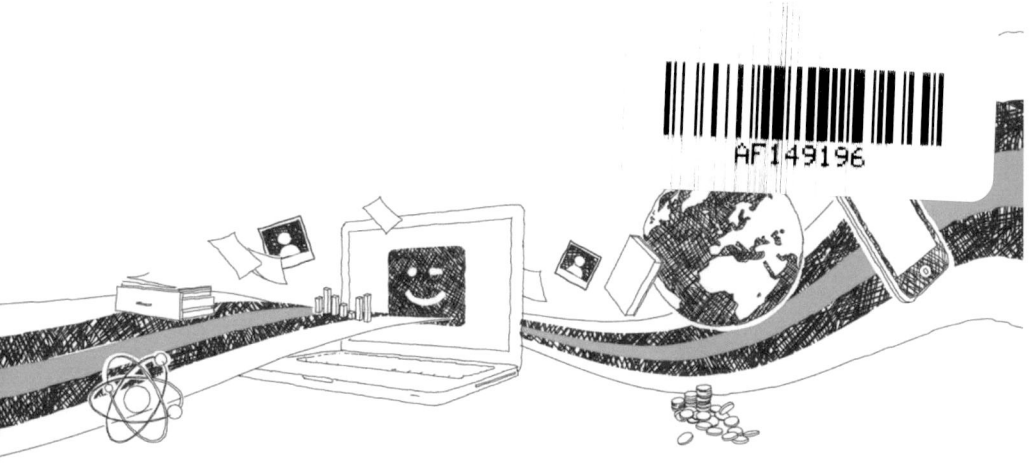

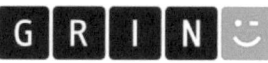

Bibliographic information published by the German National Library:

The German National Library lists this publication in the National Bibliography;
detailed bibliographic data are available on the Internet at http://dnb.dnb.de .

Imprint:

Copyright © 2016 GRIN Verlag, Open Publishing GmbH
Print and binding: Books on Demand GmbH, Norderstedt Germany
ISBN: 9783668239128

This book at GRIN:

http://www.grin.com/en/e-book/323942/reflection-and-its-uses-in-problem-solving-
and-personal-development

Kiran Kumar

Reflection and its uses in Problem Solving and Personal Development

GRIN Publishing

GRIN - Your knowledge has value

Since its foundation in 1998, GRIN has specialized in publishing academic texts by students, college teachers and other academics as e-book and printed book. The website www.grin.com is an ideal platform for presenting term papers, final papers, scientific essays, dissertations and specialist books.

Visit us on the internet:

http://www.grin.com/

http://www.facebook.com/grincom

http://www.twitter.com/grin_com

Organising Modern Healthcare Services

Reflective Writing

Table of Contents

INTRODUCTION..3

METHODOLOGY 3

Reflective Model Frame Work 5

Gibbs Model of Reflection (1988)..6

ANALYSIS..6

CONCLUSION..8

REFERENCES 9

INTRODUCTION

We learn by experiences which allow us to absorb what we read, hear and feel and help to do the activity and mainly interact with the people which help us to socialize (Wertenbroch&Nabeth, 2000). Reflection is an thinking of an extended period which are interlinked with the recent experience it also involves commonalities, differences and interrelation beyond their superficial elements (Dewey 1933) reflection is a form of problem solving that chained several ideas together by linking with its predecessor in order to resolve the issues which are raised.

According to Hatton & Smith (1995) they identified four essential issue which concern reflection That We should learn to frame and reframe complex or ambiguous problems, test out various interpretations, and then modify our actions consequently. Our thoughts should be extended and systematic by looking back upon our actions sometime after they have taken place. Certain activities labelled as reflective, such as the use of journals or group discussions following practical experiences, are often not directed towards the solution of specific problems. We should consciously account for the wider historic, cultural, and political values or beliefs in framing practical problems to arrive at a solution. This is often identified as critical reflection. However, the term critical reflection, like reflection itself, appears to be used loosely, some taking it to mean no more than constructive self-criticism of one's actions with a view to improvement.

Rationale Reflection is the conscious weighing and integrating of views from different perspectives which is a necessary prerequisite for the development of a balanced professional identity acquiring knowledge and practical skills alone are not enough to become a medical professional. 'Reflecting on education and clinical experiences in medical practice, including one's own behaviour, becomes crucial' (Boenink et al, 2004).

The reflective models used in the self-assessment are; Reflective rational Enquiry, Gibbs Reflective Cycle and Kolbs Reflective Cycle

METHODOLOGY

The reflective models used in the self-assessment is Reflective Rational Enquiry proposed by Lawrence-Wilkes&Ashmore(2014), it involves a framework for an self-improvement it helps us to assess our own thoughts and actions for the purpose of personal learning and development it can be used for our own development or others to develop the reflective practise is mainly concerned with self-development which enables us for future personal growth and how we think and feel about our self and situations in the past and present.

Reflective Enquiry

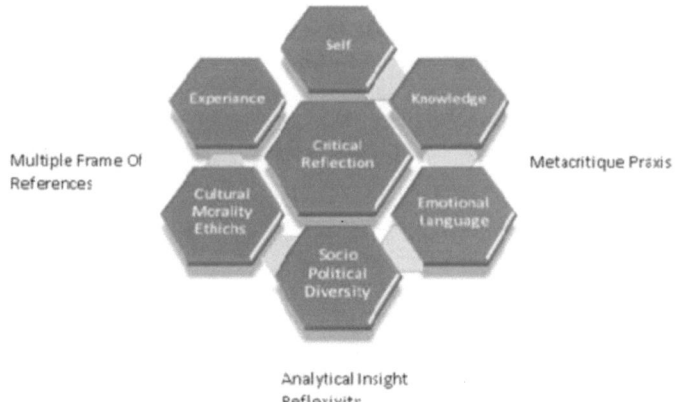

Reflective Rational Enquiry : Lawrence - Wilkes & Ashmore (2014)

This Reflective practice is a valuable methodology for using insights and learning from the past for assessing where we are now and what can we do to improve our present and future. For example this reflective report is based on the experience studying this unit organising modern health care services in MBA Hospital & Health Service Management its analysed by the overall unit reflection through this Reflective Rational Enquiry model helps to identify core learning outcomes assessed by our past and present, it is an internal appraisal process to identify the concern regarding experience which as to be an influential to overcome which can be changed for current and other circumstances.

Reflective Model Frame Work; (David Kolb-Experimental Learning)

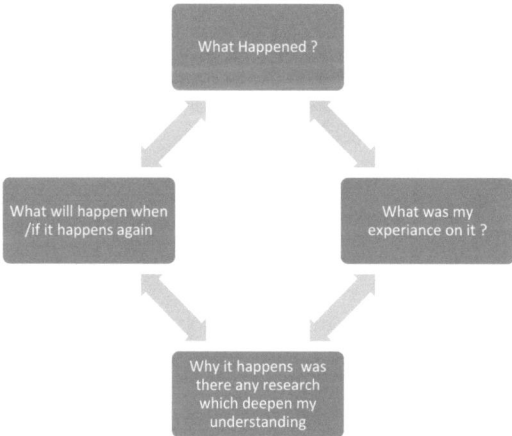

It's based on the experimental learning but was progressed to be a set of reflective prompts and an even way to structure a piece of reflective writing.

Graham Gibbs Reflective Cycle; it's a single model often applied differently academic disciples to incorporate different reflective activities. Further Gibbs model (Gibbs 1988) acts as a supportive efficient action plan it encourages the systematic thinking about the phases of experience or activity it provides an opportunity to view the various perspective on a given experience issue or action and also it helps us to have a more balanced and précised judgement.

An approach to learning and practise development which is patient centred and acknowledges the confusion of practise environment it's also gives an ability to establish a link between theory and a practise providing a rationale of actions its used to reflect once their strengths, weakness and the area of development

Gibbs reflective cycle is one of the smoothest theory to implement and begin with the reflective practises once comfortable with it will began to focus an evaluation analysis and planning phases in more detail the reflective will become even more insightfull,probing and detailed to generals the narrative description. Reflective practise is relatively remains as unknown concept in healthcare practices compared to others but some find reflective journal as a useful tool in the reflective process (Koh et al 2014; Asselin & Fain, 2013)

Gibbs Model of Reflection (1988)

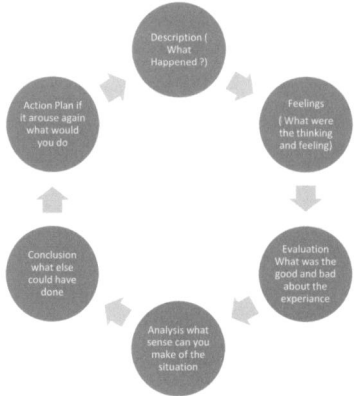

It's an efficient tool to reflect the even on critical incidents , when following this cycle it's important to ensure descriptive section, and it's one of the most relevant to this unit assessment it given an inspiration towards understanding the analytical stages of practical experience however the reflective model is supportive and directive to make an efficient action towards healthcare leadership the reasons to use this reflective methodology is to embrace myself to create an self-awareness and create an successful career ahead .Being applied to healthcare leadership it's useful as it describes the things where the leaders are doing at work and demonstrates how we can develop as a leader by overcoming our efficiency to be best suited formal leadership role.

Gibbs reflective cycle (1988) have been described with 6 stages in the cycle description ,thoughts and feelings, evaluation, analysis , conclusion and action plan it encourages with a clear and objective description ,analysis and evaluation from our own experience it also help us to lead us to some of the useful information which considers what we have learned from the experience and what might to do differently if the situation occur again its creates an response to experience, opinions and new information an response to thoughts and feelings a way of thinking to explore the learning's it creates an opportunity to gain knowledge and achieving a great clarity and a better understanding of learning and more over a way of making meaning out of what I study.

ANALYSIS

On The Basis of Proposed model of Reflective rational enquiry and reflective model frame work of Kolb experimental learning including Gibbs model of reflection it enables to review my past experiences and its helpful to support my development skills to deliver my best to my professional career way. When it comes to the unit organising modern healthcare the reflective rational model help to gain the critical reflection of being self and approach by my knowledge with the prior experience depending upon the multiple frames of reference there was much more diifentiation regarding cultural morality ethics and scio economic diversity expectancy was high , the analytical insight towards covered my thoughts has I completed my bachelors in medical laboratory technology and having about few experience in both service and managerial level its was bit convincing by self-evaluation I just wanted to develop some of the more managerial and leadership skills in management has I had some bitter experience in management I adapted the experimental learning procedure to explore myself within the career pathway the organising healthcare service really motivated to concise my practical approach towards the fact.

Below are the description of the Gibbs reflective stages individually described about the reliability and diversity of organising modern health care within the industry how it have supported during the assessment.

Description: Organising modern healthcare services is one of the most import unit for the healthcare professionals the key areas like healthcare expenditure and procurement and leadership and management in UK healthcare gives an deep immense outlook over the healthcare industry and outbreak and critical analysis of Francis report and mind mapping all this models were relatively significant in enhance in the leadership and qualitative management skills which will be an added advantage at the workplace to explore and apply our learning experience practically.

Feeling : This was the crucial stage where we need to compare the things with our past and present experiences has it was an new experience and unit there was an huge expectation to know the things presently occurring in the healthcare industry and how we can develop the leadership and managerial skills and presentation and research around the healthcare descriptive was seemingly very explorative interesting which give an satisfaction.

Evaluation:

This unit provided a structured back space to deepen and apply notions of systems working to the specific challenges of organising complex health care service of summons effectively and efficiently. The unit was designed for backing the exploration of best recitation and praxis theory practice relevant for Wellness Religious service delivery in prentice own contexts.

Appreciative query and problem based learning promote the skills of critical analytic thinking, negotiation and resolution required of all Health Care leaders. Player will be provided with scenarios for argumentation, analysis and the merits of proposed firmness will be further explored.

The teaching, learning and assessment philosophy of a clear and constructive approaching is chosen deliberately to funding participants to develop the depth of critical evaluation required to generate a study recommending responses to a specifically identified Health Care Divine service design issue, and reflect on the value of the process as a whole.

In this unit we have an guest lecture regarding leadership and management ,Francis report , conception procedure leading in teenage pregnancy and ethics and issues which are presently in NHS ex ; increased waiting period of patients all the issues and concern regarding management skills and development was an interesting fact which covered by this topic.

Analysis

In this stage was one of the crucial as we need to evaluate and analysed and does a kind of self-assessments the development of managerial skills and leadership session which were more practical rather than interactive which help us to come out with some of the leadership qualities at such circumstances I have attained some new skills through the design and evaluate and critically think on mind map and providing our analysis about the critical appraisel about the mortality statistics which can lead to improve the quality of the patient care in the hospital system

CONCLUSION

The reflective writing report on the self-assessments was really help full for assessing the knowledge and experience gained in this unit based on the proposed model of reflective rational enquiry , Kolb's experimenting learning, and Gibbs learning model delivers an incite note of the value of experience which is gained in the unit had embarked the gracious of learning in the MBA course which indeed help to know the health care management system in many organisations and changing ideas of and knowing and understanding different types of healthcare managerial skills in different countries more of the good ethical moral behaviour is learnt and the many supportive things which came across this unit can be used in further in my career pathway.

To be a good social healthcare leader the knowledge which is gained I will be used as to acquire to develop the situational leadership enable to reach the goal in desired healthcare sector and being motivated and organising myself and showing some positive attitude towards both the work and the people involved in the organisation the developed management skills used as a key point in project management and working accordingly plan and identifies the priority of the work and issues so it highlights the relevant experience to the community and working in the hospital it enacts as an successful option of level and face upwards of my career graph.

This review has sought to identify some shared themes and narratives between social mobilising and organising and recent leadership literature. It may well be that as Helen Bevan suggests the time has come for social movement thinking to be embraced as a means of large scale change within the public sector. The leadership literature suggests that this time may come more readily if lessons from the leadership literature can be digested and used to enhance this process.

REFERENCES

- Huczynski, A. and Buchanan, D.A. (2013) Organizational behaviour. Eight edn. United Kingdom: Pearson Education Limited.

- Gibbs, G. (1988) Learning by doing: A guide to teaching and learning methods. Oxford: Oxford Further Education Unit.

- Kolb, D. A. (1984). Experiential learning: Experience as the source of learning and development (Vol. 1). Englewood Cliffs, NJ: Prentice-Hall

- Lawrence-Wilkes and Ashmore, 2014:64, The Reflective Practitioner in Professional Education

- Gibbs [1988] Learning by Doing: A guide to teaching and learning methods. Further Education Unit. Oxford Polytechnic: Oxford.

- Mezirow, J. and Associates (2000) Learning as Transformation – Critical Perspectives on a Theory in Progress. San Francisco: Jossey-Bass.

- Raelin, J (2011) from leadership as practice to leaderful practice Leadership, (2011); 7 (2) pp 195-211

- Mintzberg, H. (2004) Leadership and Management Development: An Afterword. The Academy of Management Executive Vol. 18, No. 3 pp.140-142.

- Gronn, P. (2002). Distributed leadership as a unit of analysis. The Leadership Quarterly, v13, 423-451.

YOUR KNOWLEDGE HAS VALUE

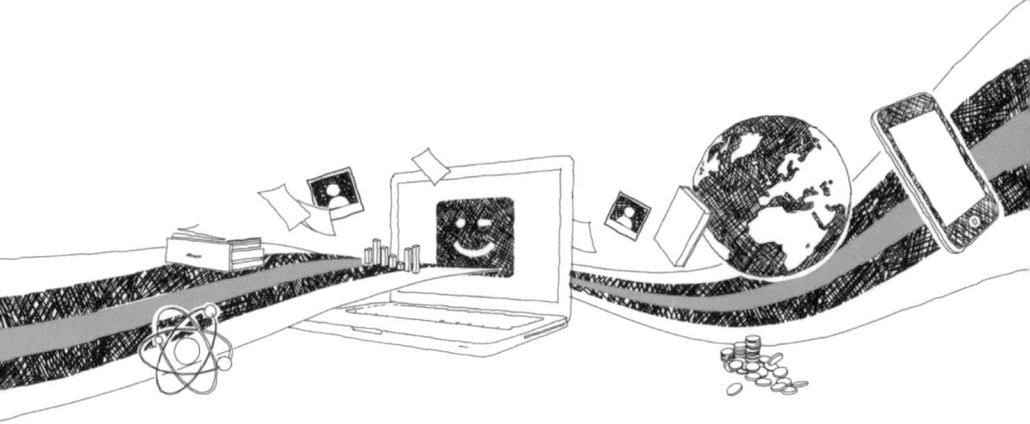

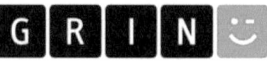